Table of Contents

CHOLESTEROL? WHAT IT MEANS AND ITS EFFECT ON YOUR HEALTH

Cholesterol is a waxy, fatty substance produced naturally by your liver and found in your blood. Cholesterol is used for many different things in your body, but it can become a problem when there is too much of it in your blood.

High levels of cholesterol in your blood are mainly caused by eating foods that aren't part of a heart-healthy eating pattern. By following a heart-healthy eating pattern, you will be eating in a way that is naturally low in unhealthy fats and high in healthy fats.

TYPES OF CHOLESTEROL

The two main types of cholesterol are:

I. Low-density lipoprotein (LDL) – also known as 'bad' cholesterol because it can add to the build-up of pla�ue (fatty deposits) in your arteries and increase your risk of coronary heart disease.

II. High-density lipoprotein (HDL) – also known as 'good' cholesterol because it can help to protect you against coronary heart disease.

HOW IS CHOLESTEROL MEASURED?

Most people with high cholesterol feel perfectly well and often have no symptoms.

Visit your GP to find out your cholesterol level (with a blood test) and to find out what you need to do if your levels of bad cholesterol are high.

WHAT CAUSES HIGH CHOLESTEROL?

Some causes of high cholesterol include:

1) High intake of foods containing unhealthy fats (saturated fats and trans fats) – such as fatty meats and deli-style meats, butter, cream, ice cream, coconut oil, palm oil and most deep-fried takeaway foods and commercially baked products (such as pies, biscuits, buns and pastries).
2) Low intake of foods containing healthy fats – healthy fats tend to increase the good

(HDL) cholesterol. Foods containing healthy fats include avocado, nuts, seeds, olives, cooking oils made from plants or seeds, and fish.

3) Low intake of foods containing fibre – foods that are high in dietary fibre, particularly soluble fibre, can reduce the amount of bad (LDL) cholesterol in your blood. Include fibre-containing foods in your diet by choosing vegetables, fruits, wholegrains, legumes, nuts and seeds every day.
4) Low levels of physical activity and exercise.
5) Being overweight or obese and having too much body fat around your middle.
6) Smoking can lead to high cholesterol levels.
7) Genetics: your family history may affect your cholesterol level. In some families, several people might be diagnosed with high cholesterol or heart disease at a relatively young age (men below age 55 years and women below 65 years). This type of pattern can be caused by genetics,

including a genetic condition called familial "hypercholesterolaemia".

8) Drinking too much alcohol can increase your cholesterol and triglyceride levels.
9) Some medical conditions can cause high cholesterol levels including kidney and liver disease and underactive thyroid gland (hypothyroidism). People with type 2 diabetes and high blood pressure often have high cholesterol.

Some types of medicines you take for other health problems can increase cholesterol levels as well.

CHOLESTEROL AND HEALTHY EATING

What we eat has an impact on our cholesterol levels and can help reduce our risk of disease. The Heart Foundation recommends following a heart-healthy eating pattern, which means eating a wide variety of fresh and unprocessed foods and limiting highly processed foods including take away, baked goods, chocolate, chips, lollies and sugary drinks. Not only does this help to maintain a healthy and interesting diet, but it provides essential nutrients to the body.

A heart-healthy eating pattern includes:

- plenty of vegetables, fruit and wholegrains
- a variety of healthy protein-rich foods (especially fish and seafood), legumes (such as beans and lentils), nuts and seeds. Smaller amounts of eggs and lean poultry can also be included in a heart-healthy eating pattern. If choosing red meat, make sure it is lean and limit to one to three times a week
- unflavoured milk, yoghurt and cheese. People with high cholesterol should choose reduced fat varieties
- healthy fats and oils. Choose nuts, seeds, avocados, olives and their oils for cooking
- herbs and spices to flavour foods, instead of adding salt.

This way of eating is also naturally high in fibre, which is good news, because a high intake of dietary fibre can also reduce levels of bad cholesterol in the blood.

Also, be mindful of how much you are eating. Portion sizes can increase over time and many of us are eating more than we need which can increase our cholesterol and risk of heart disease.

Ideally, a healthy plate would include servings of ¼ healthy proteins, ¼ wholegrains and ½ colourful vegetables.

FOODS THAT WILL HELP REDUCE YOUR CHOLESTEROL LEVELS

1. **KALE**:
   Kale is an excellent source of fiber and many other nutrients. One cup of boiled kale contains 4.7 g of fiber. Including more fiber in the diet can help lower levels of total cholesterol and LDL cholesterol. Kale is also very rich in antioxidants, which are good for the heart and help reduce inflammation.
2. **EXTRA VIRGIN OLIVE OIL**:

Extra virgin olive oil features regularly in the heart-healthy Mediterranean diet. One of its many uses is as a cooking oil. Substituting saturated fat, found in butter, with monounsaturated fat, found in extra virgin olive oil, might help reduce LDL levels. Moreover, extra virgin olive oil has antioxidant and anti-inflammatory properties that can be very beneficial to cardiovascular and overall health.

3. **GARLIC**:

   People can use garlic in a wide range of dishes, and it has many health benefits. For example, researchers have found that garlic can help regulate serum cholesterol levels. And another study determined that garlic can also help reduce blood pressure.

4. **GREEN TEA**

   Antioxidants called catechins in certain teas, such as green tea, can be very beneficial to health. Researches have shown that green tea consumption significantly improved cholesterol levels, reducing both total and LDL cholesterol levels without lowering HDL cholesterol levels.

5. **DARK CHOCOLATE**:
   Cocoa, which can be found in dark chocolate, contains flavonoids, a group of compounds in many fruits and vegetables. Their antioxidant and anti-inflammatory properties can benefit health in various ways. Some study showed participants who drank a beverage containing cocoa flavanol twice a day for a month had their LDL cholesterol levels and blood pressure had decreased, and their HDL cholesterol levels had increased. However, eat dark chocolate products in moderation, as they can be high in saturated fats and sugar.
6. **OATS**:
   Oats significantly improves blood cholesterol levels.
   It has been confirmed that the soluble fiber in oats lowers LDL cholesterol levels and can improve cardiovascular risk as part of a

heart-healthy diet. A person can add oats to their diet by eating porridge or oat-based cereal for breakfast.

7. **FISH**:

   Omega-3 fats, such as eicosapentaenoic acid (EPA), are essential polyunsaturated fats found in fish such as salmon, mackerel, and sardines, with well-documented anti-inflammatory and heart health benefits. EPA can help protect the blood vessels and heart from disease by lowering levels of triglycerides, a fat that enters the bloodstream after a meal. This is one of many ways that it may prevent atherosclerosis and reduce the risk of cardiovascular disease.

8. **BARLEY**:

   Barley is a healthy grain that is rich in vitamins and minerals and high in fiber. Beta-glucan, a type of soluble dietary fiber found in barley, as well as oats, can help lower LDL cholesterol.

The body uses cholesterol to produce bile acids, replacing those that are trapped, which leads to an overall reduction in cholesterol levels.

The beta-glucan in barley also has a positive effect on the gut microbiome and blood glucose control, further benefiting heart health.

9. **NUTS**:

   Nuts are a good source of unsaturated fats, which can help lower LDL cholesterol levels, especially when they replace saturated fats in the diet. Nuts are also rich in fiber, which helps keep the body from absorbing cholesterol and promotes its excretion. All nuts are suitable for a heart-healthy, cholesterol-lowering diet, including:

- almonds
- walnuts
- pistachios
- pecans
- hazelnuts
- Brazil nuts

- cashews

10. **AVOCADO**:

    Avocados are rich in heart-healthy nutrients. It is believed that eating one avocado a day as part of a moderate fat, cholesterol-lowering diet can improve cardiovascular disease risk, specifically by lowering LDL cholesterol without lowering HDL cholesterol. One cup, or 150 g, of avocado contains 14.7 g of monounsaturated fats, which can reduce LDL cholesterol levels and lower the risk of heart disease and strokes.

11. **APPLES**:

    A study found that among 40 participants with mildly high cholesterol, eating two apples a day reduced both total and LDL cholesterol levels. It also lowered levels of triglycerides, a type of fat in the blood. One apple can contain 3–7 g of dietary fiber, depending on its size. In addition, apples contain compounds called polyphenols, which may also have a positive impact on cholesterol levels.

12. **SOY**:

    Soybeans and soy products, such as tofu, soy milk, and soy yogurt, are suitable for a cholesterol-lowering diet.

13. **LENTILS**:

    Lentils are rich in fiber, containing 3.3 g per 100-g portion. Fiber can prevent the body from absorbing cholesterol into the bloodstream.

FOODS TO AVOID

To reduce levels of "bad" cholesterol, limit the intake of the following foods, which contain high levels of saturated and trans fats:

- fatty meat, such as lamb and pork
- lard and shortening
- butter and cream
- palm oil
- cakes and donuts
- pastries
- potato chips

- fried foods
- full fat dairy products

LOW CHOLESTEROL DIET RECIPE JUST FOR YOU

TOFU AND BROWN RICE WITH VEGGIES

INGREDIENTS:

- 500 grams orange sweet potatoes peeled and cut into cubes
- olive oil cooking spray
- 1 1/3 cups cooked brown rice
- 1 can corn kernels
- 300 grams broccoli florets
- 200 grams Chinese soy tofu cut into cubes
- 1/3 cup fresh flat-leaf parsley leaves chopped

INSTRUCTIONS:

1. Preheat oven to 400°F.
2. Get your baking pan and line it with parchment paper. Arrange the sweet potato

cubes and tofu then spray with oil. Toss lightly to coat well.

3. Bake for 30 to 35 minutes or until tender and the tofu becomes crispy.
4. In a microwave-safe bowl, place the broccoli florets and corn along with 2 tablespoons of cold water to keep it hydrated. Cover with a plastic wrap or with parchment paper and microwave on high for 4 to 5 minutes or until the broccoli is tender and bright green.
5. Rinse the broccoli under cold water and drain well.
6. In a bowl, spoon some brown rice and top it with the sweet potatoes, tofu, broccoli, and corn. Season with salt and pepper. Serve with parsley.

LOW CHOLESTEROL CHICKEN MEATLOAF

INGREDIENTS:

- 1 lb ground chicken, or any lean ground meat like chuck or turkey
- 2 cups oats, ⍰uick-cooking

- 11 oz marinara sauce, divided
- 3 oz red onion, minced
- 2 oz bell peppers, of your choice, minced
- 1½ oz carrots, minced
- salt, to taste
- ground black pepper, to taste

TO SERVE:

- 1½ cups potato, fried
- 4 oz vegetables, (green beans, onions, and tomatoes), pan-grilled
- parsley

INSTRUCTIONS:

1. Preheat the oven to 350 degrees F. Grease a loaf tin and baking sheet with cooking spray.
2. In a bowl, combine the ground chicken, 7 ounces of marinara sauce, onions, bell peppers, carrots, and oats in a bowl.
3. Season with salt and pepper, then mix all the ingredients together, then transfer into the greased loaf pan.

4. Cover with foil, then transfer to the oven. Bake for 1 hour, or until meatloaf is fully cooked.
5. Once baked, remove and discard the foil. Pour off any excess liquid or fat, then invert onto your greased baking sheet.
6. Pour over the remaining marinara sauce and spread to cover the meatloaf. Return back to the oven and broil until the sauce glazes the meatloaf.
7. Portion accordingly, serve with potatoes and vegetables done your way, then garnish with parsley. Enjoy!

MEDITERRANEAN BREAKFAST BURRATA PLATTER

INGREDIENTS:

- 2 cups butternut squash cubes
- 2 teaspoons extra virgin olive oil
- 1/4 teaspoon kosher salt
- Freshly ground black pepper
- 4 whole grain bread slices
- One 8-oz ball burrata

- 1 cup microgreens
- 2 Tbsp pumpkin seeds
- Balsamic vinegar

INSTRUCTIONS:

1. Preheat oven to 400°F. Place the butternut s⍰uash in a medium bowl, drizzle with extra virgin olive oil, and sprinkle with salt and pepper. Toss to coat. Spread out in a single layer on a lined baking sheet. Roast butternut s⍰uash for 30 to 35 minutes, flipping s⍰uash halfway through. S⍰uash is ready when fork tender and lightly browned in some areas.
2. Toast the bread. Cut slices in half and place on a large platter with burrata and butternut squash. Top with microgreens, pumpkin seeds, and a drizzle of balsamic vinegar.

HEALTHY OATMEAL WITH PEANUT BUTTER AND BANANA

INGREDIENTS:

- 4 1/2 cups water
- 2 cups rolled oats
- Pinch of salt
- 2 bananas, sliced
- 2 Tbsp peanut butter
- 1/4 cup chopped almonds
- 2 Tbsp agave syrup

INSTRUCTIONS:

1. In a medium saucepan, bring the water to a boil. Turn the heat down to low and add the oatmeal and salt. Cook, stirring occasionally, for about 5 minutes, until the oats are tender and have absorbed most of the liquid.
2. Add the bananas, peanut butter, almonds, and agave syrup and stir to incorporate evenly. If the oatmeal is too thick, add a splash of milk.

SPECIAL BANANA BREAD

INGREDIENT:

- 4 very ripe bananas, peeled and mashed (about 2 cups)
- 1/2 cup Greek-style yogurt
- 4 Tbsp butter, melted
- 2 large eggs
- tsp vanilla
- cups flour
- 3/4 cup sugar
- 1/2 cup toasted walnuts, coarsely chopped
- 1 tsp baking soda
- 1 tsp baking powder
- 1/2 tsp ground cinnamon
- 1/2 tsp salt

INSTRUCTIONS:

1. Preheat the oven to 350°F. Butter a 9" x 5" x 3" loaf pan.
2. Combine the bananas, yogurt, butter, eggs, and vanilla in a large mixing bowl, stirring to blend. In a separate bowl, mix together the flour, sugar, walnuts, baking soda, baking

powder, cinnamon, and salt. Gently fold the dry ingredients into the wet banana mixture, and stir until fully incorporated.

3. Scrape the batter into the prepared pan.
4. Bake on a low oven rack for about 50 minutes, until a toothpick inserted into the center of the bread comes out clean. Let cool for 5 minutes in the pan.
5. Eat warm or at room temperature.

DESSERT-WORTHY FRUIT AND GRANOLA YOGURT PARFAIT RECIPE

INGREDIENTS:

- cup sliced strawberries (you can also use juicy fruit like raspberries, blackberries, kiwi, and mangoes.)
- 1⁄2 cup blueberries (frozen are good, too)
- tsp sugar
- 4–5 mint leaves, sliced thinly
- 1 container (8 oz) low-fat plain Greek-style yogurt (If you don't dig the thick Greek yogurt, any plain yogurt will work, as long as there are no added sugars.)

- 1⁄4 cup granola

INSTRUCTIONS:

1. Combine the fruit, sugar, and mint in a bowl, and allow to sit for 3 to 4 minutes.
2. Spoon half of the yogurt into a bowl or glass, then top with half of the fruit and granola, then repeat with the remaining yogurt, fruit, and granola.
3. Pour any accumulated juice from the fruit over the top.

BREAKFAST VEGGIE BURGER

INGREDIENTS

- Field Roast veggie
- burger patty
- thick slice tomato
- thin slices red onion
- 1/4 avocado, sliced
- tsp canola oil
- large egg
- Freshly ground black pepper
- Fresh parsley

INSTRUCTIONS:

1. Heat a cast-iron skillet over medium heat. Cook the patty on each side for about 3 minutes until browned. Place the tomato slice on a plate, and top it with sliced onion and the veggie patty.
2. Heat oil in a non-stick skillet over medium-low heat. Gently crack the egg into the skillet. Cook low and slow until the white is completely set, about 3 to 5 minutes.
3. Top the burger with the egg. Add black pepper and parsley. Serve with avocado on the side.

HEALTHY TURKEY CHILI

INGREDIENTS:

- 2 teaspoons olive oil
- yellow onion, chopped
- garlic cloves, minced
- 1 medium red bell pepper, chopped
- 1 pound extra lean ground turkey or chicken

- 2 tablespoons chili powder
- 2 teaspoons ground cumin
- 1 teaspoon dried oregano
- 1/4 teaspoon cayenne pepper
- 1/2 teaspoon salt, plus more to taste
- 1 (28-ounce) can diced tomatoes or crushed tomatoes
- 1 1/4 cups chicken broth
- 2 (15 oz) cans dark red kidney beans, rinsed and drained
- 1 (15 oz) can sweet corn, rinsed and drained

FOR TOPPING:

- cheese, avocado, tortilla chips, cilantro, sour cream

INSTRUCTIONS:

1. Place oil in a large pot and place over medium high heat. Add in onion, garlic and red pepper and saute for 5-7 minutes, stirring frequently.
2. Add in ground turkey and break up the meat; cooking until no longer pink. Next

add in chili powder, cumin, oregano, cayenne pepper and salt; stir for about 20 seconds.

3. Next add in tomatoes, chicken broth, kidney beans and corn. Bring to a boil, then reduce heat and simmer for 30-45 minutes or until chili thickens and flavors come together. Taste and adjust seasonings and salt as necessary.
4. Garnish with anything you'd like.

AIR FRYER EGG WHITE FRITTATA

INGREDIENTS:

- 2 cups li�uid egg whites
- 1/2 cup chopped fresh spinach
- 1/4 cup chopped Roma tomato
- 1/2 teaspoon salt
- 1/4 cup chopped white onion

INSTRUCTIONS:

1. Preheat the air fryer to 320 degrees F. Spray a 6" round baking dish with cooking spray.

2. In a large bowl, whisk egg whites until frothy. Mix in spinach, tomato, salt, and onion. Stir until combined.
3. Pour egg mixture into prepared dish.
4. Place in the air fryer basket and cook 8 minutes until the center is set. Serve warm.

CHICKPEA QUINOA SOUP

INGREDIENTS:

- tablespoon canola oil.
- 1 cup sliced halved carrots
- 1 cup chopped yellow bell pepper
- 1/2 cup chopped onion
- cloves garlic, minced
- 1 32-ounce carton unsalted vegetable stock or reduced-sodium vegetable broth
- 1 14.5-ounce can no-salt-added
- petite diced or diced tomatoes, undrained
- 1 8-ounce can of no-salt-added tomato sauce
- 1 15-ounce can no-salt-added chickpeas, rinsed and drained

- 1/3 cup uncooked □uinoa, rinsed and drained
- 1 tablespoon Worcestershire sauce
- teaspoon chili powder
- 1 teaspoon dried oregano, crushed
- 1 teaspoon ground cumin
- 1/2 teaspoon salt
- 1/4 teaspoon black pepper
- 1 medium zucchini, quartered lengthwise and sliced (1 1/3 cups)
- Light sour cream, shredded reduced-fat cheddar cheese, and/or chopped fresh cilantro

INSTRUCTIONS:

1. In a oven, heat oil over medium-high. Add carrots, bell pepper, onion, and garlic; cook and stir 4 minutes.
2. Carefully add the next 11 ingredients (from vegetable stock to black pepper). Bring to boiling; reduce heat. Cover and simmer 20 minutes or until carrots are just tender.

3. Add zucchini; cook 5 to 7 minutes more or until crisp-tender. top each serving with sour cream, cheese, and/or cilantro.

SNICKERDOODLE PROTEIN MINI MUFFINS

INGREDIENTS:

- 3/4 cup Vanilla Tone It Up Protein
- 3/4 cup almond meal
- 2 tsp. cinnamon
- tsp. baking powder
- 1/4 tsp. salt
- 1 egg
- 1 tsp. vanilla extract
- 1/2 cup dates, pitted and soaked in warm water to soften
- 3/4 cup unsweetened almond milk
- 1 mashed banana
- Coconut oil spray

INSTRUCTIONS:

1. Preheat oven to 350 degrees.
2. Combine all dry ingredients in a bowl.

3. Combine all wet ingredients, including the dates, in a blender, and blend until smooth. Add wet ingredients to the dry ingredients and mix to combine.
4. Spray a mini muffin tin with coconut oil spray. Pour batter into the muffin tins.
5. Bake for 20-25 minutes or until a toothpick comes out clean.
6. Top with a little extra sprinkle of cinnamon.

EASY CHICKEN CASSEROLE

INGREDIENTS:

- 2 tbsp sunflower oil
- 400g boneless, skinless chicken thigh , trimmed and cut into chunks
- 1 onion , finely chopped
- 3 carrots , finely chopped
- 3 celery sticks, finely chopped
- 2 thyme sprigs or ½ tsp dried
- 1 bay leaf , fresh or dried
- 600ml vegetable or chicken stock
- 2 x 400g / 14oz cans haricot beans , drained
- chopped parsley , to serve

INSTRUCTIONS:

1. Heat the oil in a large pan, add the chicken, then fry until lightly browned. Add the veg, then fry for a few mins more. Stir in the herbs and stock. Bring to the boil. Stir well, reduce the heat, then cover and cook for 40 mins, until the chicken is tender.
2. Stir the beans into the pan, then simmer for 5 mins. Stir in the parsley and serve with crusty bread.

SUMMER VEGETABLE CURRY

INGREDIENTS:

- 1-2 tbsp red Thai curry paste (how you like it)
- 500ml low-sodium vegetable stock
- 2 onions , chopped
- 1 aubergine , diced
- 75g red lentil
- 200ml can reduced-fat coconut milk
- 2 red or yellow peppers , deseeded and cut into wedges
- 140g frozen pea

- 100g bag baby spinach , roughly chopped
- brown basmati rice and mango chutney, to serve

INSTRUCTIONS:

1. Heat the curry paste in a large non-stick saucepan with a splash of the stock. Add the onions and fry for 5 mins until starting to soften. Stir in the aubergine and cook for a further 5 mins – add a little more stock if starting to stick.
2. Add the lentils, coconut milk and the rest of the stock, and simmer for 15 mins or until the lentils are tender. Add the peppers and cook for 5-10 mins more. Stir through the peas and spinach and cook until spinach has just wilted. Serve the curry with rice and mango chutney.

VEGAN TAGINE

INGREDIENTS:

- 2 tbsp olive oil
- 2 onions , chopped

- ½ tsp each ground cinnamon , coriander and cumin
- 2 large courgettes , cut into chunks
- 2 chopped tomatoes
- 400g can chickpea , rinsed and drained
- 4 tbsp raisin
- 425ml vegetable stock
- 300g frozen pea
- chopped coriander , to serve

INSTRUCTIONS:

1. Heat the oil in a pan, then fry the onions for 5 mins until soft. Stir in the spices. Add the courgettes, tomatoes, chickpeas, raisins and stock, then bring to the boil. Cover and simmer for 10 mins. Stir in the peas and cook for 5 mins more. Sprinkle with coriander, to serve.

TROUT EN PAPILLOTE

INGREDIENTS:

- 2 large carrots , cut into batons
- 3 celery sticks, cut into batons

- 1 tbsp olive oil
- ½ tsp sugar
- 6 tbsp white wine vinegar
- 4 x 175g trout fillets
- basil leaves
- juice 1 lemon

INSTRUCTIONS:

1. Heat oven to 190C/fan 170C/gas 5. Put the carrots and celery in a pan with the oil, sugar, wine, salt and pepper. Bring to the boil, tightly cover, then cook for 10 mins until the vegetables are tender. Cool.
2. Cut four large sheets of baking parchment, about 35cm s□uare. Divide the vegetables between them and top each with a trout fillet. Scatter a few basil leaves and a little lemon juice over each, then season the fish with a little salt and pepper. Fold the paper in half and double fold all round to seal in the fish, a bit like a pasty.
3. Put the parcels on two baking sheets and bake for 15-20 mins (depending on the

thickness of the fish). Serve in their paper with some steamed new potatoes.

SALMON & SPINACH WITH TARTARE CREAM

INGREDIENTS:

- 1 tsp sunflower or vegetable oil
- 2 skinless salmon fillets
- 250g bag spinach
- 2 tbsp reduced-fat crème fraîche
- juice ½ lemon
- 1 tsp caper, drained
- 2 tbsp flat-leaf parsley, chopped
- lemon wedges, to serve

INSTRUCTIONS:

1. Heat the oil in a pan, season the salmon on both sides, then fry for 4 mins each side until golden and the flesh flakes easily. Leave to rest on a plate while you cook the spinach.
2. Tip the leaves into the hot pan, season well, then cover and leave to wilt for 1 min,

stirring once or twice. Spoon the spinach onto plates, then top with the salmon. Gently heat the crème fraîche in the pan with a s⍰ueeze of the lemon juice, the capers and parsley, then season to taste. Be careful not to let it boil. Spoon the sauce over the fish, then serve with lemon wedges.

INDIAN WINTER SOUP

INGREDIENTS:

- 100g pearl barley
- 2 tbsp vegetable oil
- ½ tsp brown mustard seeds
- 1 tsp cumin seeds
- 2 green chillies, deseeded and finely chopped
- 1 bay leaf
- 2 cloves
- 1 small cinnamon stick
- ½ tsp ground turmeric
- 1 large onion, chopped
- 2 garlic cloves, finely chopped

- 1 parsnip, cut into chunks
- 200g butternut squash, cut into chunks
- 200g sweet potato, cut into chunks
- 1 tsp paprika
- 1 tsp ground coriander
- 225g red lentils
- 2 tomatoes, chopped
- small bunch coriander, chopped
- 1 tsp grated ginger
- 1 tsp lemon juice

INSTRUCTIONS:

1. Rinse the pearl barley and cook following pack instructions. When it is tender, drain and set aside. Meanwhile, heat the oil in a deep, heavy-bottomed pan. Fry the mustard seeds, cumin seeds, chillies, bay leaf, cloves, cinnamon and turmeric until fragrant and the seeds start to crackle. Tip in the onion and garlic, then cook for 5-8 mins until soft. Stir in the parsnip, butternut and sweet potato and mix thoroughly, making sure the vegetables are fully coated with the oil and spices. Sprinkle in the

paprika, ground coriander and seasoning, and stir again.

2. Add the lentils, pearl barley, tomatoes and 1.7 litres water. Bring to the boil then turn down and simmer until the vegetables are tender. When the lentils are almost cooked, stir in the chopped coriander, ginger and lemon juice.

SQUASH & BARLEY SALAD WITH BALSAMIC VINAIGRETTE

INGREDIENTS:

- 1 butternut s?uash , peeled and cut into long pieces
- 1 tbsp olive oil
- 250g pearl barley
- 300g Tenderstem broccoli , cut into medium-size pieces
- 100g SunBlush tomato , sliced
- 1 small red onion , diced
- 2 tbsp pumpkin seeds
- 1 tbsp small capers , rinsed
- 15 black olives , pitted

- 20g pack basil , chopped

FOR THE DRESSING:

- 5 tbsp balsamic vinegar
- 6 tbsp extra-virgin olive oil
- 1 tbsp Dijon mustard
- 1 garlic clove , finely chopped

INSTRUCTIONS:

1. Heat oven to 200C/fan 180C/gas 6. Place the s�uash on a baking tray and toss with olive oil. Roast for 20 mins. Meanwhile, boil the barley for about 25 mins in salted water until tender, but al dente. While this is happening, whisk the dressing ingredients in a small bowl, then season with salt and pepper. Drain the barley, then tip it into a bowl and pour over the dressing. Mix well and let it cool.
2. Boil the broccoli in salted water until just tender, then drain and rinse in cold water. Drain and pat dry. Add the broccoli and remaining ingredients to the barley and mix

well. Can be left for 3 days in the fridge and is delicious warm or cold.

SEEDED OATCAKES

INGREDIENTS:

- 50g butter
- 100g medium oatmeal
- 100g plain flour , plus extra for dusting
- 1 tsp bicarbonate of soda
- 2 tsp poppy seed
- 2 tbsp sesame seed

INSTRUCTIONS:

1. Heat oven to 200C/180C fan/gas 6. Melt the butter in a small pan, then allow to cool slightly. Tip all the dry ingredients into a bowl, with ½ tsp salt, then pour in the butter. Add 5-6 tbsp boiling water and combine to make a firm dough.
2. Turn out the dough onto a lightly floured surface, then roll out until about 0.5cm thick. Cut into small s�uares, then bake for 12-15 mins until golden. Leave to cool for a

few mins, then transfer to a wire rack and cool completely.

LOW-FAT MOUSSAKA

INGREDIENTS:

- 200g frozen sliced peppers
- 3 garlic cloves , crushed
- 200g extra-lean minced beef
- 100g red lentils
- 2 tsp dried oregano , plus extra for sprinkling
- 500ml carton passata
- 1 aubergine , sliced into 1.5cm rounds
- 4 tomatoes , sliced into 1cm rounds
- 2 tsp olive oil
- 25g parmesan , finely grated
- 170g pot 0% fat Greek yogurt
- freshly grated nutmeg

INSTRUCTIONS:

1. Cook the peppers gently in a large non-stick pan for about 5 mins – the water from them should stop them sticking. Add the garlic

and cook for 1 min more, then add the beef, breaking up with a fork, and cook until brown. Tip in the lentils, half the oregano, the passata and a splash of water. Simmer for 15-20 mins until the lentils are tender, adding more water if you need to.

2. Meanwhile, heat the grill to Medium. Arrange the aubergine and tomato slices on a non-stick baking tray and brush with the oil. Sprinkle with the remaining oregano and some seasoning, then grill for 1-2 mins each side until lightly charred – you may need to do this in batches.
3. Mix half the Parmesan with the yogurt and some seasoning. Divide the beef mixture between 4 small ovenproof dishes and top with the sliced aubergine and tomato. Spoon over the yogurt topping and sprinkle with the extra oregano, Parmesan and nutmeg. Grill for 3-4 mins until bubbling.

NOODLES WITH TURKEY, GREEN BEANS & HOISIN

INGREDIENTS:

- 100g ramen noodles
- 100g green beans , halved
- 3 tbsp hoisin sauce
- juice 1 lime
- 1 tbsp chilli sauce
- 1 tbsp vegetable oil
- 250g turkey mince
- 2 garlic cloves , chopped
- 6 spring onions , sliced diagonally

INSTRUCTIONS:

1. Boil the noodles following pack instructions, adding the green beans for the final 2 mins. Drain and set aside.
2. In a small bowl, mix together the hoisin, lime juice and chilli sauce. In a wok or frying pan, heat the oil, then fry the mince until nicely browned. Add the garlic and fry for 1 min more. Stir in the hoisin mixture and cook for a few mins more until sticky.

Finally, stir in the noodles, beans and half the spring onions to heat through. Scatter over the remaining spring onions to serve.

CINNAMON PORRIDGE WITH BANANA & BERRIES

INGREDIENTS:

- 100g porridge oats
- ½ tsp cinnamon , plus extra to serve
- 4 tsp demerara sugar
- 450ml skimmed milk
- 3 bananas , sliced
- 400g punnet strawberries , hulled and halved
- 150g pot fat-free natural yogurt

INSTRUCTIONS:

1. In a medium-sized saucepan, mix the oats, cinnamon, sugar, milk and half the sliced bananas. Bring to the boil, stirring occasionally. Turn down the heat and cook for 4-5 mins, stirring all the time.

2. Remove and divide between 4 bowls, top with the remaining banana, strawberries, a dollop of yogurt and a sprinkle of cinnamon.

SPICED CHICKEN WITH RICE & CRISP RED ONIONS

INGREDIENTS:

- 2 boneless skinless chicken breasts, about 140g/5oz each
- 1 tbsp sunflower oil
- 2 tsp curry powder
- 1 large red onion , thinly sliced
- 100g basmati rice
- 1 cinnamon stick
- pinch saffron
- 1 tbsp raisins
- 85g frozen pea
- 1 tbsp chopped mint and coriander
- 4 rounded tbsp low-fat natural yogurt

INSTRUCTIONS:

1. Heat oven to 190C/fan 170C/gas 5. Brush the chicken with 1 tsp oil, then sprinkle with

curry powder. Toss the onion in the remaining oil. Put the chicken and onions in one layer in a roasting tin. Bake for 25 mins until the meat is cooked and the onions are crisp, stirring the onions halfway through the cooking time.

2. Rinse the rice, then put in a pan with the cinnamon, saffron, salt to taste and 300ml water. Bring to the boil, stir once, add the raisins, cover. Gently cook for 10-12 mins until the rice is tender, adding the peas halfway through. Spoon the rice onto two plates, top with the chicken and scatter over the onions. Stir the herbs into the yogurt and season, if you like, before serving on the side.

POTATO CURRY WITH ROTI

INGREDIENTS:

- 600g desiree potatoes, peeled, cut into 1cm-thick slices
- tbsp vegetable oil
- 1 red onion, thinly sliced

- garlic cloves, thinly sliced
- 6cm piece fresh ginger, finely grated
- 1 tsp yellow mustard seeds
- 1 tsp cumin seeds
- tsp ground coriander
- 1/2 tsp ground turmeric
- roti
- 1/3 cup low-fat Greek-style yoghurt
- 1/2 cup fresh coriander sprigs
- Mango chilli chutney, to serve
- Coriander sprigs, extra, to serve

INSTRUCTIONS:

1. Cook potato in a large saucepan of boiling salted water for 2 to 3 minutes or until just tender. Drain.
2. Heat oil in a large frying pan over high heat. Add onion, garlic and ginger. Cook, stirring, for 3 minutes or until softened. Stir in seeds, ground coriander and turmeric. Cook, stirring, for 1 minute or until fragrant.

3. Add potato and 1/2 cup cold water. Cook for 2 to 3 minutes or until potato is tender and water has evaporated.
4. Meanwhile, heat roti following packet directions. Place roti on serving plates. Cover half of each roti with potato filling. Dollop with yoghurt and top with coriander. Fold roti over to cover filling. Serve with chutney and sprinkled with extra coriander.

SPICED CHICKEN WITH RICE & CRISP RED ONIONS

INGREDIENTS:

- 2 boneless skinless chicken breasts, about 140g/5oz each
- 1 tbsp sunflower oil
- 2 tsp curry powder
- 1 large red onion , thinly sliced
- 100g basmati rice
- 1 cinnamon stick
- pinch saffron
- 1 tbsp raisins
- 85g frozen pea

- 1 tbsp chopped mint and coriander
- 4 rounded tbsp low-fat natural yogurt

INSTRUCTIONS:

1. Heat oven to 190C/fan 170C/gas 5. Brush the chicken with 1 tsp oil, then sprinkle with curry powder. Toss the onion in the remaining oil. Put the chicken and onions in one layer in a roasting tin. Bake for 25 mins until the meat is cooked and the onions are crisp, stirring the onions halfway through the cooking time.
2. Rinse the rice, then put in a pan with the cinnamon, saffron, salt to taste and 300ml water. Bring to the boil, stir once, add the raisins, cover. Gently cook for 10-12 mins until the rice is tender, adding the peas halfway through. Spoon the rice onto two plates, top with the chicken and scatter over the onions. Stir the herbs into the yogurt and season, if you like, before serving on the side.

OPEN SANDWICHES - CRUSHED BEAN, ARTICHOKE & RED ONION

INGREDIENTS:

- 1 slice granary bread
- 1 small can haricot bean
- basil oil
- artichoke heart , from a jar
- sundried tomatoes , from a jar
- few slices red onion

INSTRUCTIONS:

1. Toast a slice of bread.
2. Drain the haricot beans and mash in a bowl with a little oil. Season if you like.
3. Spoon over the toast and top with artichoke hearts and sundried tomatoes, a few slices red onion and a little more oil, if you like.

CRAB LINGUINE WITH CHILLI & PARSLEY

INGREDIENTS:

- 400g linguine
- 4 tbsp extra-virgin olive oil

- 1 red chilli, deseeded and chopped
- 2 garlic cloves, finely chopped
- 1 whole cooked crab, picked, or about 100g/4oz brown crabmeat and 200g/7oz fresh white crabmeat
- small splash, about 5 tbsp, white wine
- small s⍰ueeze of lemon (optional)
- large handful flat-leaf parsley leaves, very finely chopped

INSTRUCTIONS:

1. Bring a large pan of salted water to the boil and add the linguine. Give it a good stir and boil for 1 min less than the pack says. Stir well occasionally so it doesn't stick.
2. While the pasta cooks, gently heat 3 tbsp of olive oil with the chilli and garlic in a pan large enough to hold all the pasta comfortably. Cook the chilli and garlic very gently until they start to sizzle, then turn up the heat and add the white wine. Simmer everything until the wine and olive oil come together. Then take off the heat and add the brown crabmeat, using a wooden

spatula or spoon to mash it into the olive oil to make a thick sauce.

3. When the pasta has had its cooking time, taste a strand – it should have a very slight bite. When it's ready, turn off the heat. Place the sauce on a very low heat and use a pair of kitchen tongs to lift the pasta from the water into the sauce.
4. Off the heat, add the white crabmeat and parsley to the pasta with a sprinkling of sea salt. Stir everything together really well, adding a drop of pasta water if it's starting to get claggy. Taste for seasoning and, if it needs a slight lift, add a small squeeze of lemon. Serve immediately twirled into pasta bowls and drizzled with the remaining oil.

SPAGHETTI WITH SARDINES

INGREDIENTS:

- 400g spaghetti
- tbsp olive oil
- garlic cloves , crushed
- pinch chilli flakes

- 227g can chopped tomato
- x cans skinless and boneless sardines in tomato sauce
- 100g pitted black olives , roughly chopped
- 1 tbsp capers , drained
- small handful parsley , chopped

INSTRUCTIONS:

1. Cook the spaghetti in a large pan of boiling salted water according to pack instructions. Meanwhile, make the sauce. Heat the oil in a medium pan and cook the garlic for 1 min. Add the chilli flakes, tomatoes and sardines, breaking up roughly with a wooden spoon. Heat for 2-3 mins, then stir in the olives, capers and most of the parsley. Mix well to combine.
2. Drain the pasta, reserving a couple of tbsp of the water. Add the pasta to the sauce and mix well, adding the reserved water if the sauce is a little thick. Divide between 4 bowls and sprinkle with the remaining parsley.

DEVILLED TOFU KEBABS

INGREDIENTS:

- 8 shallots or button onions
- 8 small new potatoes
- 2 tbsp tomato purée
- 2 tbsp light soy sauce
- 1 tbsp sunflower oil
- 1 tbsp clear honey
- 1 tbsp wholegrain mustard
- 300g firm smoked tofu , cubed
- 1 courgette , peeled and sliced
- 1 red pepper , deseeded and diced

INSTRUCTIONS:

1. Put the shallots or button onions in a bowl, cover with boiling water and set aside for 5 mins. Cook the potatoes in a pan of boiling water for 7 mins until tender. Drain and pat dry. Put tomato purée, soy sauce, oil, honey, mustard and seasoning in a bowl, then mix well. Toss the tofu in the marinade. Set aside for at least 10 mins.

2. Heat the grill. Drain and peel shallots or onions, then cook in boiling water for 3 mins. Drain well. Thread the tofu, shallots, potatoes, courgette and pepper on to 8 x 20cm skewers. Grill for 10 mins, turning fre�uently and brushing with remaining marinade before serving.

MANDARIN, ASPARAGUS AND BABY BEETROOT SALAD

INGREDIENTS:

- 4 (1 bunch) baby beetroot, trimmed
- 3 mandarins
- 1/2 tbsp extra virgin olive oil
- bunches asparagus, trimmed, cut into 4cm lengths
- 120g baby rocket
- 1/2 cup crunchy combo sprouts, rinsed
- 50g low-fat feta, crumbled

INSTRUCTIONS:

1. Preheat oven to 200C/180C fan-forced. Wash beetroot and pat dry. Place in a

baking dish. Cover tightly with foil. Roast for 40 to 45 minutes or until skin peels away from beetroot when rubbed. Set aside until cool enough to handle.

2. Wearing rubber gloves, peel and halve each beetroot, ⍰uartering any larger ones.
3. Juice 1 mandarin (1/4 cup juice). Place juice in a bowl. Add oil. Season with salt and pepper. Whisk to combine.
4. Place asparagus in a heatproof bowl. Cover with boiling water. Stand for 4 minutes or until bright green and tender. Drain. Peel remaining mandarins, removing all the white pith, and divide into segments. Place rocket on a platter. Top with beetroot, asparagus, mandarin, sprouts and fetta. Drizzle with dressing. Serve.

CARROT AND BEETROOT SLAW WITH FENNEL DRESSING

INGREDIENTS:

- 4 large carrots

- 4 beetroot (300g each), washed, trimmed, peeled
- 1/4 cup pecans, roughly chopped
- 2 tbsp sultanas
- 2 cups fresh flat-leaf parsley leaves
- Fennel dressing
- 1/2 tsp fennel seeds
- tsp Dijon mustard
- 1/4 cup apple cider vinegar
- 1 1/2 tbsp extra virgin olive oil

INSTRUCTIONS:

1. Make Fennel dressing: Place fennel seeds in a mortar. Pound with a pestle until crushed. Whisk mustard, crushed fennel seeds, vinegar and oil together in a small bowl. Season with salt and pepper.
2. Using the grater attachment on a food processor, coarsely grate carrot. Transfer to a bowl. Continue process with beetroot, placing in a separate bowl to the carrot.
3. Add pecans, sultanas and parsley to carrot. Pour over dressing. Toss until well

combined. Add beetroot, Gently toss to combine. Serve.

CHARGRILLED TURKEY WITH ?UINOA TABBOULEH & TAHINI DRESSING

INGREDIENTS:

- 200g ?uinoa
- ½ cucumber , cut into 1cm chunks
- 175g cherry tomato , halved
- 3 spring onions , finely sliced
- handful parsley , roughly chopped
- handful coriander , roughly chopped
- 1 tbsp olive oil , plus 1 tsp
- juice 1 lemon
- 4 turkey steaks

FOR THE TAHINI DRESSING

- 1½ tbsp tahini paste
- 1½ tbsp low-fat yogurt
- juice ½ lemon
- ½ garlic clove, crushed
- ½ tsp clear honey

INSTRUCTIONS:

1. Tip the quinoa into a saucepan and pour over 600ml water. Cover with a lid and bring to the boil. Turn down and simmer until the water has evaporated (about 20 mins. Take off the lid and leave to cool while you prepare the turkey and salad.
2. Tip the cucumber, tomatoes, spring onions and herbs into a large mixing bowl. Pour over 1 tbsp olive oil and lemon juice, season well and mix everything together.
3. Heat a griddle pan and, when smoking hot, rub the turkey steaks with 1 tsp olive oil. Cook for about 5 mins on each side, depending on thickness. Stir together all the dressing ingredients along with 3 tbsp water. Toss the ⍰uinoa together with the salad and arrange on plates. Cut the turkey into thick slices, pile up on the ⍰uinoa and drizzle over the dressing.

CANNELLINI BEAN AND TOMATO SALAD

INGREDIENTS:

- 400g can cannellini beans, drained, rinsed
- 1/2 small red onion, finely chopped
- 200g grape tomatoes, halved
- 2 tbsp red wine vinegar
- tbsp olive oil

INSTRUCTIONS:

1. Combine beans , onion and tomato in a large bowl. Add vinegar and oil . Toss to combine. Cover with plastic wrap. Stand for 30 minutes for flavours to develop. Serve.

PORK SKEWERS WITH BURGHUL SALAD

INGREDIENTS:

- 500g extra-trim pork loin steaks, cut into 2cm cubes
- tbsp Middle Eastern seasoning
- 500g eggplant, cut into 2cm cubes
- 1 large red capsicum, cut into 2cm cubes
- 300g zucchini, cut into 2cm cubes

- 500g jap pumpkin, peeled, cut into 2cm cubes
- olive oil cooking spray
- 1/2 cup burghul (cracked wheat)
- 1 cup boiling water
- tbsp chopped fresh flat-leaf parsley leaves
- tbsp chopped fresh coriander leaves
- 1 1/2 tbsp fat-free Italian dressing
- lemon wedges, to serve

INSTRUCTIONS:

1. Preheat oven to 220°C/200°C fan-forced. Line 2 roasting trays with baking paper.
2. Place pork and seasoning in a shallow glass or ceramic dish. Stir to coat. Thread pork onto skewers. Cover and refrigerate.
3. Divide eggplant , capsicum , zucchini and pumpkin between prepared trays. Spray with oil . Roast for 30 to 40 minutes or until tender and light golden.
4. Meanwhile, place burghul in a large, heatproof bowl. Cover with boiling water . Set aside for 10 minutes. Drain. Using

hands, s⍰ueeze out excess li⍰uid. Return to bowl.

5. Spray a barbecue plate or chargrill with oil. Heat over medium heat. Cook skewers for 2 minutes each side or until cooked through.
6. Add roasted vegetables, parsley , coriander and dressing to burghul. Season with salt and pepper. Toss to combine. Serve skewers with burghul mixture and lemon wedges .

KIDNEY BEAN CURRY

INGREDIENTS:

- 1 tbsp vegetable oil
- 1 onion, finely chopped
- 2 garlic cloves, finely chopped
- thumb-sized piece of ginger, peeled and finely chopped
- 1 small pack coriander, stalks finely chopped, leaves roughly shredded
- 1 tsp ground cumin
- 1 tsp ground paprika
- 2 tsp garam masala

- 400g can chopped tomatoes
- 400g can kidney beans, in water
- cooked basmati rice, to serve

INSTRUCTIONS:

1. Heat the oil in a large frying pan over a low-medium heat. Add the onion and a pinch of salt and cook slowly, stirring occasionally, until softened and just starting to colour. Add the garlic, ginger and coriander stalks and cook for a further 2 mins, until fragrant.
2. Add the spices to the pan and cook for another 1 min, by which point everything should smell aromatic. Tip in the chopped tomatoes and kidney beans in their water, then bring to the boil.
3. Turn down the heat and simmer for 15 mins until the curry is nice and thick. Season to taste, then serve with the basmati rice and the coriander leaves.

PUTTANESCA BAKED GNOCCHI

INGREDIENTS:

- 2 x 400g cans cherry tomatoes
- olive oil, for frying
- 1 onion, finely chopped
- 1 tsp chilli flakes
- 1 tbsp capers, drained
- 60g black pitted Kalamata olives, roughly chopped
- 5 anchovy fillets in oil, finely chopped
- pinch of sugar
- 500g shop-bought gnocchi
- 1 x 125g ball mozzarella, torn

INSTRUCTIONS:

1. Blitz one of the cans of tomatoes until smooth and set aside. Heat a glug of oil in a medium-sized saucepan over a medium heat. Add the onion and a generous pinch of salt and fry gently for 8-10 mins until softened and translucent. Tip the chilli and all the tomatoes into the pan, lower the heat, then simmer for 10 mins, uncovered.

Fill one of the empty cans a quarter full with water and add this to the sauce. Stir through the capers, olives and anchovies. Season with salt, pepper and a couple of generous pinches of sugar. Cook on a gentle heat, uncovered, for a further 5 mins. Keep warm until needed.

2. Bring a large pan of water to the boil. Add the gnocchi and cook for 2 mins. Drain and toss with the tomato sauce, then tip into an ovenproof dish or shallow casserole. Top with the torn mozzarella and a good grating of black pepper then pop under a high grill for 3-4 mins or until the mozzarella is molten and gooey.

CHICKEN & MUSHROOM HOT-POT

INGREDIENTS:

- 50g butter or margarine, plus extra for greasing
- 1 onion, chopped
- 100g button mushrooms, sliced
- 40g plain flour

- 1 chicken stock cube or 500ml fresh chicken stock
- pinch of nutmeg
- pinch of mustard powder
- 250g cooked chicken, chopped
- 2 handfuls of a mixed pack of sweetcorn, peas, broccoli and carrots, or pick your favourites

FOR THE TOPPING

- 2 large potatoes, sliced into rounds
- knob of butter, melted

INSTRUCTIONS:

1. Heat oven to 200C/180C fan/gas 6. Put the butter in a medium-size saucepan and place over a medium heat. Add the onion and leave to cook for 5 mins, stirring occasionally. Add the mushrooms to the saucepan with the onions.
2. Once the onion and mushrooms are almost cooked, stir in the flour – this will make a thick paste called a roux. If you are using a stock cube, crumble the cube into the roux

now and stir well. Put the roux over a low heat and stir continuously for 2 mins – this will cook the flour and stop the sauce from having a floury taste.

3. Take the roux off the heat. Slowly add the fresh stock, if using, or pour in 500ml water if you’ve used a stock cube, stirring all the time. Once all the li�uid has been added, season with pepper, a pinch of nutmeg and mustard powder. Put the saucepan back onto a medium heat and slowly bring it to the boil, stirring all the time. Once the sauce has thickened, place on a very low heat. Add the cooked chicken and vegetables to the sauce and stir well. Grease a medium-size ovenproof pie dish with a little butter and pour in the chicken and mushroom filling.
4. Carefully lay the potatoes on top of the hot-pot filling, overlapping them slightly, almost like a pie top.
5. Brush the potatoes with a little melted butter and cook in the oven for about 35

mins. The hot-pot is ready once the potatoes are cooked and golden brown.

EDAMAME & CHILLI DIP WITH CRUDITÉS

INGREDIENTS:

- 300g frozen soya bean
- 150g low-fat natural yogurt
- 1 red chilli , chopped
- juice 1 lime
- 1 garlic clove , crushed
- 1 red onion , finely chopped
- handful coriander , chopped
- halved radishes , sticks of carrots, celery and peppers, to serve

INSTRUCTIONS:

1. Cook the soya beans in boiling salted water for 4 mins. Drain and cool under cold running water. Blitz with the yogurt, chopped red chilli, lime juice and crushed garlic clove until smooth. Fold in the finely chopped red onion and a handful chopped coriander. Serve with halved radishes and

sticks of carrots, celery and peppers. The dip will keep covered in the fridge for up to 3 days.

CHILD-FRIENDLY THAI CHICKEN NOODLES

INGREDIENTS:

- 100g sugar snap peas
- 1 tbsp oil
- 2 spring onions , finely chopped
- 2 garlic cloves , crushed
- 1 tsp grated ginger
- 3 x chicken breasts, cut into chunks
- 1-1 ½ tbsp Thai curry paste
- 400ml can coconut milk
- 2 limes , juice of one, other ⍰uartered
- 50g frozen peas
- 3 nests egg noodles
- handful chopped coriander , to serve

INSTRUCTIONS:

2. Blanch the sugar snap peas in a bowl of boiling water for 2 mins, then drain. Heat the oil in a large frying pan. Add the spring

onions, garlic, ginger and chicken. Gently fry for 2-3 mins. Stir in the curry paste and cook for 1 minute more. Add the coconut milk to the pan, along with a splash of water, the lime juice, peas and sugar snap peas. Gently bubble for around 5 mins until the chicken is cooked through.

3. Meanwhile, cook the noodles according to the pack instructions. Drain. Stir the noodles through the sauce, scatter with coriander and serve with a wedge of lime for squeezing over.

SWEET POTATO & PEANUT CURRY

INGREDIENTS:

- 1 tbsp coconut oil
- 1 onion, chopped
- 2 garlic cloves, grated
- thumb-sized piece ginger, grated
- 3 tbsp Thai red curry paste (check the label to make sure it's vegetarian/ vegan)
- 1 tbsp smooth peanut butter

- 500g sweet potato, peeled and cut into chunks
- 400ml can coconut milk
- 200g bag spinach
- 1 lime, juiced
- cooked rice, to serve (optional)
- dry roasted peanuts, to serve (optional)

INSTRUCTIONS:

1. Melt 1 tbsp coconut oil in a saucepan over a medium heat and soften 1 chopped onion for 5 mins. Add 2 grated garlic cloves and a grated thumb-sized piece of ginger, and cook for 1 min until fragrant.
2. Stir in 3 tbsp Thai red curry paste, 1 tbsp smooth peanut butter and 500g sweet potato, peeled and cut into chunks, then add 400ml coconut milk and 200ml water.
3. Bring to the boil, turn down the heat and simmer, uncovered, for 25-30 mins or until the sweet potato is soft.
4. Stir through 200g spinach and the juice of 1 lime, and season well. Serve with cooked

rice, and if you want some crunch, sprinkle over a few dry roasted peanuts.

FISH PIE MAC 'N' CHEESE

INGREDIENTS:

- 650ml milk
- 40g plain flour
- 40g butter
- 2 tsp Dijon mustard
- 150g mature cheddar , grated
- 180g frozen peas
- handful of parsley , chopped
- 300g macaroni
- 300g fish pie mix (smoked fish, white fish and salmon)
- green salad , to serve (optional)

INSTRUCTIONS:

1. Pour the milk into a large pan and add the flour and butter. Set over a medium heat and whisk continuously until you have a smooth, thick white sauce. Remove from the heat, add the mustard, most of the

cheese (save some for the top), peas and parsley.

2. Meanwhile, boil the pasta in a large pan of water following pack instructions until just cooked. Drain.
3. Heat the oven to 200C/180C fan/gas 6. Tip the pasta into the sauce and add half the fish, stir everything together then tip into a large baking dish. Top with the rest of the fish, pushing it into the pasta a little, then scatter with the remaining cheese. Bake for 30 mins until golden, then serve with salad, if you like. Can be chilled and eaten within three days or frozen for up to a month.

EASY CARROT CAKE

INGREDIENTS:

- 230ml vegetable oil, plus extra for the tin
- 100g natural yogurt
- 4 large eggs
- 1½ tsp vanilla extract
- ½ orange, zested
- 265g self-raising flour

- 335g light muscovado sugar
- 2½ tsp ground cinnamon
- ¼ fresh nutmeg, finely grated
- 265g carrots (about 3), grated
- 100g sultanas or raisins
- 100g walnuts or pecans, roughly chopped

FOR THE ICING

- 100g slightly salted butter, softened
- 300g icing sugar
- 100g soft cheese

INSTRUCTIONS:

1. Heat the oven to 180C/160C fan/gas 4. Oil and line the base and sides of two 20cm cake tins with baking parchment. Whisk the oil, yogurt, eggs, vanilla and zest in a jug. Mix the flour, sugar, cinnamon and nutmeg with a good pinch of salt in a bowl. S�ueeze any lumps of sugar through your fingers, shaking the bowl a few times to bring the lumps to the surface.
2. Add the wet ingredients to the dry, along with the carrots, raisins and half the nuts, if

using. Mix well to combine, then divide between the tins.

3. Bake for 25-30 mins or until a skewer inserted into the centre of the cake comes out clean. If any wet mixture clings to the skewer, return to the oven for 5 mins, then check again. Leave to cool in the tins.
4. To make the icing, beat the butter and sugar together until smooth. Add half the soft cheese and beat again, then add the rest (adding it bit by bit prevents the icing from splitting). Remove the cakes from the tins and sandwich together with half the icing. Top with the remaining icing and scatter with the remaining walnuts. can kept in the fridge for up to five days.

SLOW COOKER HONEY MUSTARD CHICKEN THIGHS

INGREDIENTS:

- 1 tbsp butter
- 8 chicken thighs
- 8 spring onions, cut into lengths

- 150ml chicken stock
- 1 tbsp Dijon mustard
- 2 tbsp honey
- 2 tbsp double cream or crème fraîche
- 100g frozen peas

INSTRUCTIONS:

1. Heat the slow cooker. Melt the butter in a frying pan and □uickly brown the chicken thighs all over. Make sure the skin picks up plenty of colour. Season, then put them in the slow cooker. Brown the spring onions and add them to the slow cooker as well. Add the stock, mustard and honey and cook on low for 4 hrs.
2. Stir in the cream or crème fraîche and peas, then cook for a further 15 mins with the lid off. Re-crisp up the chicken skin under the grill, if you like.

SAVOY CABBAGE WITH ALMONDS

INGREDIENTS:

- 1 Savoy cabbage , finely sliced

- 25g butter
- 1 tbsp olive oil
- 1 garlic clove , sliced
- 1 rosemary sprig, leaves finely chopped
- 100g blanched almond

INSTRUCTIONS:

1. Steam or microwave the cabbage until just cooked. Melt the butter with the oil in a large frying pan or wok, then add the garlic, rosemary and almonds. Cook, stirring the almonds for about 2 mins or until they start to brown. Tip onto a plate. Add the cabbage to the pan, stir in the leftover buttery juices, then return the almond mixture to the pan. Season well and tip into a serving dish.

SAUSAGE RAGU

INGREDIENTS:

- 3 tbsp olive oil
- 1 onion, finely chopped
- 2 large garlic cloves, crushed
- ¼ tsp chilli flakes

- 2 rosemary sprigs, leaves finely chopped
- 2 x 400g cans chopped tomatoes
- 1 tbsp brown sugar
- 6 pork sausages
- 150ml whole milk
- 1 lemon, zested
- 350g rigatoni pasta
- grated parmesan and ½ small bunch parsley, leaves roughly chopped, to serve

INSTRUCTIONS:

1. Heat 2 tbsp of the oil in a saucepan over a medium heat. Fry the onion with a pinch of salt for 7 mins. Add the garlic, chilli and rosemary, and cook for 1 min more. Tip in the tomatoes and sugar, and simmer for 20 mins.
2. Heat the remaining oil in a medium frying pan over a medium heat. Squeeze the sausagemeat from the skins and fry, breaking it up with a wooden spoon, for 5-7 mins until golden. Add to the sauce with the milk and lemon zest, then simmer for a further 5 mins. To freeze, leave to cool

completely and transfer to large freezerproof bags.

3. Cook the pasta following pack instructions. Drain and toss with the sauce. Scatter over the parmesan and parsley leaves to serve.

VEGETABLE TAGINE WITH APRICOTS

INGREDIENTS:

- 2 tsp olive oil
- brown onion, halved, cut into wedges
- carrots, peeled, coarsely chopped
- garlic cloves, crushed
- 2 tsp finely grated fresh ginger
- 2 tsp cumin seeds
- 2 tsp ground paprika
- 1 x 7cm cinnamon stick
- Large pinch of saffron threads
- 375ml (1 1/2 cups) Massel vegetable liquid stock
- 650g butternut pumpkin, deseeded, peeled, coarsely chopped
- 250g green beans, topped, cut into 6cm lengths

- 100g dried Turkish apricots
- 100g fresh dates, halved, pitted
- 1 x 400g can chickpeas, rinsed, drained
- 2 tsp finely grated lemon rind
- 1/3 cup fresh coriander leaves
- Greek-style natural yoghurt, to serve

INSTRUCTIONS:

1. Heat oil in a saucepan over medium heat. Add onion and cook, stirring, for 5 minutes or until soft. Add the carrot , garlic , ginger , cumin seeds , paprika , cinnamon and saffron and cook, stirring, for 30 seconds or until aromatic.
2. Add stock and bring to the boil. Add the pumpkin , beans and apricots . Reduce heat to medium and cook, stirring occasionally, for 15 minutes or until the pumpkin is tender. Add dates , chickpeas and lemon rind and stir to combine.
3. Spoon among serving bowls and top with coriander . Serve with yoghurt .

FISH STEW

INGREDIENTS:

- tbsp extra-light olive oil
- 4 garlic cloves, finely chopped
- 1 tsp ground turmeric
- x 400g cans whole peeled tomatoes
- 400g can cannellini beans, drained, rinsed
- 600g ling fish fillets, cut into large pieces
- 1/3 cup fresh coriander leaves, chopped
- crusty wholegrain bread rolls, to serve

INSTRUCTIONS:

1. Heat oil in a large saucepan over medium heat. Add garlic . Cook, stirring, for 1 minute. Add turmeric . Cook, stirring, for 30 seconds. Reduce heat to low. Stir in tomatoes and 1 cup of cold water. Cover and bring to the boil. Simmer, covered, for 10 minutes.
2. Add beans and return to the boil. Add fish . Cover and cook for 5 minutes or until fish is cooked through.

3. portion stew into bowls and sprinkle with coriander . Serve with bread rolls .

ROAST BEEF AND ROCKET WRAP

INGREDIENTS:

- x 400g can chickpeas, rinsed, drained
- 1 tbsp tahini
- 1 garlic clove, chopped
- tbsp fresh lemon juice
- 1/2 tsp ground cumin
- pieces wholemeal lavash bread
- 250g sliced rare roast beef
- 200g (1 cup) 97 per cent fat-free semi-dried tomatoes, chopped
- 1 bunch rocket, stems trimmed, washed, dried

INSTRUCTIONS:

1. Place chickpeas , tahini , garlic , lemon juice and cumin in the bowl of a food processor and process until smooth.
2. Place the lavash on a clean work surface. Spread evenly with chickpea mixture, and

top with roast beef , semi-dried tomato and rocket .

3. Roll up lavash to enclose filling. Cut in half diagonally and serve immediately.

MARINATED TOFU AND SHIITAKE MUSHROOM STIR FRY

INGREDIENTS:

- 300g firm tofu, cut into thin strips
- 60ml (1/4 cup) mirin (rice wine)
- 2 tbsp salt-reduced soy sauce
- 2 tsp finely grated fresh ginger
- tsp caster sugar
- Vegetable oil spray
- 1 red onion, cut into thin wedges
- 150g shiitake mushrooms, halved
- bunches broccolini, ends trimmed, cut into 2cm lengths
- 1 red capsicum, deseeded, thinly sliced
- 1 tsp sesame seeds
- Steamed Basmati rice, to serve

INSTRUCTIONS:

1. Place the tofu in a shallow glass or ceramic dish. Combine half the mirin, soy sauce and ginger in a jug and pour over the tofu. Cover with plastic wrap and place in the fridge for 30 minutes to marinate.
2. Combine the sugar and remaining mirin, soy sauce and ginger in a small bowl. Heat a wok or frying pan over high heat. Lightly spray with olive oil spray. Drain the tofu and reserve the marinade. Add one-third of the tofu to the wok and cook for 1-2 minutes each side or until golden brown. Transfer to a plate. Repeat, in 2 more batches, with the remaining tofu.
3. Lightly spray the wok with olive oil spray. Add the onion and stir-fry for 1 minute or until brown. Add the mushroom and stir-fry for 1-2 minutes or until tender. Add the broccolini and capsicum and stir-fry for 1 minute or until almost tender. Add the tofu, mirin mixture and reserved marinade and stir-fry for 1-2 minutes or until broccolini is

tender crisp and the marinade comes to the boil.

4. Divide the rice among serving bowls. Top with the stir-fry and sprinkle with sesame seeds to serve.

BAKED FISH ON VEGETABLES

INGREDIENTS:

- 2 zucchinis, cut into wedges
- 2 red onions, cut into wedges
- 3 tomatoes, cut into wedges
- 1/4 cup pitted black olives
- 1/4 cup (60ml) olive oil
- 4 x 180g thick skinless white fish fillets (such as ling)
- small garlic clove, crushed
- 1 tbsp lemon juice
- 1 tbsp Dijon mustard
- 1/2 cup roughly chopped flat-leaf parsley

INSTRUCTIONS:

1. Preheat the oven to 200°C.

2. Toss the zucchini , onion , tomato and olives with 1 tablespoon of the oil in a baking dish. Brush another tablespoon of oil over the fish and place on the vegetables. Place in the oven and bake for 25-30 minutes until cooked through.
3. Whisk together the garlic , lemon juice , mustard and remaining oil to make a dressing.
4. Divide the cooked vegetables among plates and top each with a piece of fish.
5. Drizzle the fish with the dressing and scatter with chopped parsley .

CHICKPEA AND COUSCOUS FILLED CAPSICUM

INGREDIENTS:

- 2 large (600g) red capsicums, halved, deseeded
- 3 tsp olive oil
- 140g (2/3 cup) couscous
- 310ml (1 1/4 cups) boiling water
- brown onion, chopped

- 1 300g can chickpeas, rinsed, drained
- 85g (1/2 cup) chopped dried pitted dates
- 1/2 tsp ground ginger
- 1/4 tsp cayenne pepper
- 1/4 tsp salt
- 1/3 cup loosely packed chopped fresh continental parsley
- 1 200g container natural set yoghurt, 99.8% fat free

INSTRUCTIONS:

1. Preheat oven to 220°C. Brush capsicums with 1 teaspoon of oil. Place, cut-side up, in roasting pan lined with foil. Roast for 10 minutes or until tender.
2. Meanwhile, place couscous in a heatproof bowl and pour over boiling water, stirring with a fork. Cover, set aside for 5 minutes or until liquid is absorbed. Fluff with fork. Heat remaining oil in a non-stick frying pan over high heat. Cook onion, stirring, for 5-6 minutes or until brown. Reduce heat to medium, add couscous, chickpeas, dates,

ginger, pepper and salt. Cook, stirring, for 2-3 minutes or until combined. Add parsley.

3. Remove capsicum from oven. Spoon couscous mixture into each half. Bake for 12-15 minutes or until brown. Serve with the yoghurt.

ULTIMATE FISH PIE

INGREDIENTS:

- 500ml semi-skimmed milk
- 3 tbsp cornflour
- 100g cooked prawns in their shells
- several thyme sprigs, preferably lemon thyme
- 2 bay leaves
- 1 garlic clove , thinly sliced
- 750g new potatoes , such as Charlotte (no need to peel)
- 1 medium leek , thinly sliced (175g prepared weight)
- 400g skinned haddock fillet
- 350g skinned salmon fillet
- 175g skinned smoked haddock fillet

- 125g tub low-fat soft cheese with garlic & herbs
- 2 tbsp finely chopped parsley
- 2 tbsp olive oil
- 2 tbsp snipped chives

INSTRUCTIONS:

1. Mix 3 tbsp of the milk into the cornflour and set aside. Pour the rest of the milk into a saucepan. Shell the prawns, reserve the meat, then drop the shells and heads (wash them first if necessary) into the milk along with the thyme sprigs, bay leaves, garlic and a grind of pepper. Bring to a boil, then remove from the heat and leave to infuse for 20 mins.
2. Meanwhile, put the potatoes into a large pan of water, bring to the boil and simmer for 20 mins until tender. Drain. Steam the sliced leek for 3 mins, then remove from the heat and set aside.
3. Strain the infused milk through a sieve into a large shallow sauté pan. Lay all the fish fillets (not the prawns) in the milk. Bring to

a boil, then lower the heat and simmer gently for 3 mins. Remove from the heat and leave, covered, for 5 mins. Use a slotted spoon to transfer all the fish to a dish and leave to cool slightly. Heat oven to 200C/180C fan/gas 6.

4. Stir the slackened cornflour, then stir it into the hot milk in the sauté pan. Return the pan to the heat and stir until thickened. Briefly stir in the soft cheese, remove from the heat, then add the parsley and season with black pepper. Stir in any li⍰uid that has drained from the fish. Break the fish into big pieces as you lay them in a 2-litre ovenproof dish so that the different varieties are evenly distributed. Scatter over the prawns and leek, then season with pepper. Pour the sauce over and give a few gentle stirs to evenly distribute the sauce and combine everything without breaking up the fish.
5. Using a large fork, crush the potatoes by breaking them up (not mashing them) into chunky pieces. Mix in the oil, chives and a

grind of black pepper. Spoon the potato crush over the fish. Sit the dish on a baking sheet and bake for 25-30 mins, or until the sauce is bubbling and the potatoes golden. Alternatively, make the dish completely, refrigerate it for several hrs or overnight, then bake at the same temperature as above for 45 mins.

OPEN SANDWICHES - CRUSHED BEAN, ARTICHOKE & RED ONION

INGREDIENTS:

- 1 slice granary bread
- 1 small can haricot bean
- basil oil
- artichoke heart , from a jar
- sundried tomatoes , from a jar
- few slices red onion

INSTRUCTIONS:

1. Toast a slice of bread.
2. Drain the haricot beans and mash in a bowl with a little oil. Season if you like.

3. Spoon over the toast and top with artichoke hearts and sundried tomatoes, a few slices red onion and a little more oil should do.

BROWN RICE, ROAST PUMPKIN AND SEED SALAD

INGREDIENTS:

- Olive oil spray, to grease
- 1kg kent pumpkin, peeled, deseeded, cut into 2-3cm pieces
- 400g (2 cups) long-grain brown rice
- 60g (1/3 cup) pepitas (pumpkin seed kernels)
- 55g (1/3 cup) sunflower seed kernels
- 80ml (1/3 cup) fresh lime juice
- tbsp soy sauce
- 1/2 tsp sesame oil
- 1 small garlic clove, crushed
- 1/4 tsp brown sugar
- 1 bunch rocket, washed, trimmed, leaves torn

INSTRUCTIONS:

1. Preheat oven to 200°C. Spray a large baking tray with olive oil to lightly grease. Arrange the pumpkin, in a single layer, on the prepared tray and spray lightly with olive oil. Bake in preheated oven, turning halfway through cooking, for 30 minutes or until light brown and tender. Remove from oven and set aside for 15 minutes to cool to room temperature.
2. Meanwhile: cook the rice in a large saucepan of boiling water for 30 minutes or until tender (do not overcook). Drain in a large colander and set aside for 30 minutes to cool to room temperature.
3. Reduce oven temperature to 180°C. Spread the pepitas and sunflower seed kernels over a large baking tray. Bake in oven, stirring halfway through cooking, for 5 minutes or until lightly toasted. Remove from oven and set aside to cool slightly.
4. Combine the lime juice, soy sauce, sesame oil, garlic and sugar in a small jug. Place the

rice in a large bowl. Drizzle with lime-juice mixture and use a large metal spoon to gently stir until well combined. Add the rocket, pumpkin, pepitas and sunflower seed kernels to the rice mixture and gently stir until well combined. Spoon salad among serving plates and serve immediately.

RED FRUIT SALAD WITH MINT SYRUP

INGREDIENTS:

- 1/3 cup caster sugar
- 10 large mint leaves
- 250g strawberries, hulled, halved
- 125g fresh raspberries
- 400g watermelon, rind removed, cut into 2.5cm cubes

INSTRUCTIONS:

1. Place sugar and 1/2 cup warm water in a small saucepan over low heat. Cook, stirring, for 3 minutes or until sugar is dissolved. Add 8 mint leaves. Increase heat to medium. Simmer, without stirring, for 8

minutes or until mixture thickens. Remove mint leaves and discard. Set mixture aside to cool.

2. Finely shred remaining mint. Place strawberries, raspberries and watermelon in a large bowl. Toss to combine. Divide between bowls. Drizzle with sugar syrup. Sprinkle with shredded mint. Serve.

SLOW-COOKER BEEF STEW

INGREDIENTS:

- 1 onion, chopped
- 2 celery sticks, finely chopped
- 2 tbsp rapeseed oil
- 3 carrots, halved and cut into chunks
- 2 bay leaves
- ½ pack thyme
- 2 tbsp tomato purée
- 2 tbsp Worcestershire sauce
- 2 beef stock cubes or stock pots
- 900g beef for braising such as skirt, buy a whole piece and cut it yourself for bigger chunks or buy ready-diced

- 2 tsp cornflour (optional)
- ½ small bunch parsley, chopped
- buttery mash, to serve (optional)

INSTRUCTIONS:

1. Fry the onion and celery in 1 tbsp oil over a low heat until they start to soften – about 5 mins. Add the carrots, bay and thyme, fry for 2 mins, stir in the purée and Worcestershire sauce, add 600ml boiling water, stir and tip everything into a slow cooker. Crumble over the stock cubes or add the stock pots and stir, then season with pepper (don't add salt as the stock may be salty).
2. Clean out the frying pan and fry the beef in the remaining oil in batches until it is well browned, then tip each batch into the slow cooker. Cook on low for 8-10 hrs, or on high for 4 hrs.
3. If you want to thicken the gravy, mix the cornflour with a splash of cold water to make a paste, then stir in 2 tbsp of the liquid from the slow cooker. Tip back into

the slow cooker, stir and cook for a further 30 mins on high. Stir in the parsley and season again to taste. Serve with mash, if you like. Leave to cool before freezing.

BOSTON BAKED BEANS

INGREDIENTS:

- 500g pack dried haricot beans
- 2 onions , roughly chopped
- 2 celery sticks, roughly chopped
- 2 carrots , roughly chopped
- 2 tbsp Dijon mustard
- 2 tbsp light muscovado sugar
- ½ tbsp black treacle or molasses
- 2 tbsp tomato purée
- 800g piece pork belly
- handful parsley , roughly chopped

INSTRUCTIONS:

1. Soak the beans in a large bowl of cold water for at least 4 hrs or overnight. Heat oven to 180C/160C fan/gas 4. Drain and rinse the beans and put in a large flameproof

casserole with 1.5 litres water. Boil for 10 mins, skimming off any scum that appears on the surface.

2. Add the onion, celery, carrot, Dijon mustard, sugar, treacle or molasses and tomato purée. Stir until everything is well mixed, then bury the piece of pork in among the beans. Cover tightly and cook in the oven for 2-2½ hrs until the beans and pork are very tender. Check halfway through the cooking time and top up with hot water from the kettle if necessary.
3. Take the pork out of the pot. Cut into large chunks and serve with the beans, sprinkled with parsley.

FRUITY OAT SLICE

INGREDIENTS:

- 150g dried apricots
- 100g dried apple
- 2 passionfruit, halved
- 2 tbsp lemon juice
- 1/2 cup rolled oats

- 1/2 cup slivered almonds, toasted
- 1/4 cup pumpkin seeds (pepitas)
- 2 tbsp linseed

TOPPING

- 75g dark chocolate, chopped
- 1/2 tsp vegetable oil

INSTRUCTIONS:

1. Grease and line a 3cm-deep, 19cm x 29cm (base) slice pan with baking paper, allowing a 2cm overhang on both long ends.
2. Place apricots , apple , passionfruit pulp and lemon juice in a food processor. Process until just smooth. Transfer to a large bowl. Process oats , almonds , pumpkin seeds and linseed until it resembles fine breadcrumbs. Add to fruit mixture. Stir to combine. Press mixture firmly into prepared pan. Refrigerate, covered, for 1 hour or until slice is firm.
3. Line a tray with baking paper. Using a serrated knife, cut slice into 16 rectangular pieces. Place on prepared tray.

4. Make topping: Place chocolate and oil in a heatproof, microwave-safe bowl. Microwave on high (100%) for 1 1/2 to 2 minutes, stirring every 30 seconds with a metal spoon, or until melted and smooth. Spoon chocolate into a snap-lock bag. Snip off 1 corner and pipe chocolate over slice. Refrigerate until firm. Wrap in plastic wrap before packing into lunchboxes.

COUSCOUS WITH SPICY SUNFLOWER SEEDS

INGREDIENTS:

- 1/2 cups couscous
- 1 1/2 cups boiling water
- 1 tbsp olive oil
- 1 tsp ground fennel seeds
- 1 tsp ground cumin
- 1/2 tsp ground turmeric
- 1/3 cup sunflower seeds
- 1 long red chilli, deseeded, thinly sliced
- 60g baby rocket
- 100g cherry tomatoes, halved

INSTRUCTIONS:

1. Place couscous and boiling water in a large, heatproof bowl. Stand, covered, for 4 to 5 minutes or until water is absorbed. Stir with a fork to separate grains.
2. Meanwhile, heat oil in a large frying pan over medium-low heat. Add fennel , cumin , turmeric and sunflower seeds . Cook, stirring, for 2 to 3 minutes or until seeds are coated. Remove from heat.
3. Add chilli , rocket , tomato and couscous to pan. Gently toss to combine. Serve.

VINTAGE CHOCOLATE CHIP COOKIES

INGREDIENTS:

- 150g salted butter, softened
- 80g light brown muscovado sugar
- 80g granulated sugar
- 2 tsp vanilla extract
- 1 large egg
- 225g plain flour
- ½ tsp bicarbonate of soda
- ¼ tsp salt

- 200g plain chocolate chips or chunks

INSTRUCTIONS:

1. Heat the oven to 190C/fan170C/gas 5 and line two baking sheets with non-stick baking paper.
2. Put 150g softened salted butter, 80g light brown muscovado sugar and 80g granulated sugar into a bowl and beat until creamy.
3. Beat in 2 tsp vanilla extract and 1 large egg.
4. Sift 225g plain flour, ½ tsp bicarbonate of soda and ¼ tsp salt into the bowl and mix it in with a wooden spoon.
5. Add 200g plain chocolate chips or chunks and stir well.
6. Use a teaspoon to make small scoops of the mixture, spacing them well apart on the baking trays. This mixture should make about 30 cookies.
7. Bake for 8–10 mins until they are light brown on the edges and still slightly soft in the centre if you press them.

8. Leave on the tray for a couple of mins to set and then lift onto a cooling rack.

WATERCRESS MASHED POTATO

INGREDIENTS:

- 650g floury potato , cut into chunks
- 100ml milk
- 25g butter
- 170g bag watercress

INSTRUCTIONS:

1. Cook the potatoes in a large pan of salted water for 15 mins or until tender. Drain well, then return to the pan to steam-dry for a few mins before mashing.
2. Push the potatoes to one side and add the milk and butter to the other side of the pan. Heat gently until the butter melts, then stir into the potatoes with the watercress and some seasoning.

COTTAGE PIE

INGREDIENTS:

- 3 tbsp olive oil
- 1¼kg beef mince
- 2 onions, finely chopped
- 3 carrots, chopped
- 3 celery sticks, chopped
- 2 garlic cloves, finely chopped
- 3 tbsp plain flour
- 1 tbsp tomato purée
- large glass of red wine (optional)
- 850ml beef stock
- 4 tbsp Worcestershire sauce
- a few thyme sprigs
- 2 bay leaves
- For the mash
- 1.8kg potatoes, chopped
- 225ml milk
- 25g butter
- 200g strong cheddar, grated
- freshly grated nutmeg

INSTRUCTIONS:

1. Heat 1 tbsp olive oil in a large saucepan and fry 1¼kg beef mince until browned – you may need to do this in batches. Set aside as it browns.
2. Put the other 2 tbsp olive oil into the pan, add 2 finely chopped onions, 3 chopped carrots and 3 chopped celery sticks and cook on a gentle heat until soft, about 20 mins.
3. Add 2 finely chopped garlic cloves, 3 tbsp plain flour and 1 tbsp tomato purée, increase the heat and cook for a few mins, then return the beef to the pan.
4. Pour over a large glass of red wine, if using, and boil to reduce it slightly before adding the 850ml beef stock, 4 tbsp Worcestershire sauce, a few thyme sprigs and 2 bay leaves.
5. Bring to a simmer and cook, uncovered, for 45 mins. By this time the gravy should be thick and coating the meat. Check after about 30 mins – if a lot of liquid remains,

increase the heat slightly to reduce the gravy a little. Season well, then discard the bay leaves and thyme stalks.

6. Meanwhile, make the mash. In a large saucepan, cover the 1.8kg potatoes which you've peeled and chopped, in salted cold water, bring to the boil and simmer until tender.
7. Drain well, then allow to steam-dry for a few mins. Mash well with the 225ml milk, 25g butter, and three-�uarters of the 200g strong cheddar cheese, then season with freshly grated nutmeg and some salt and pepper.
8. Spoon the meat into 2 ovenproof dishes. Pipe or spoon on the mash to cover. Sprinkle on the remaining cheese.
9. If eating straight away, heat oven to 220C/200C fan/gas 7 and cook for 25-30 mins, or until the topping is golden.
10. If you want to use a slow cooker, brown your mince in batches then tip into your slow cooker and stir in the vegetables, flour,

purée, wine, stock, Worcestershire sauce and herbs with some seasoning. Cover and cook on High for 4-5 hours. Make the mash following the previous steps, and then oven cook in the same way to finish.

FIVE-SPICE VEGETABLE STIR-FRY

INGREDIENTS:

- 1/2 tsp cornflour
- tbsp light soy sauce
- tbsp Chinese rice wine or dry sherry
- 1 tsp caster sugar
- 2 tsp five-spice powder
- 1 tbsp vegetable oil
- 2 red capsicums, thinly sliced
- 1 yellow capsicum, thinly sliced
- 2 bunches broccolini, trimmed, halved on the diagonal
- 200g fresh shiitake mushrooms*, thinly sliced
- 1 1/4 cups (275g) white medium-grain rice, steamed, to serve

INSTRUCTIONS:

1. Combine cornfl our and 1/3 cup (80ml) cold water in a bowl. Add soy sauce, Chinese rice wine, sugar and fi ve-spice, and mix well. Meanwhile, heat the oil in a wok over high heat until smoking.
2. Add the vegetables and stir-fry for 2 minutes. Add sauce mixture and stir-fry for 2 minutes or until vegetables have softened but are still crunchy, and sauce has thickened.
3. Divide the stir-fry among serving plates and serve with steamed rice.

CAJUN MUSHROOMS

INGREDIENTS:

- tbsp olive oil
- 500g cup mushrooms, �uartered
- 1/2 tsp dried chilli flakes
- garlic cloves, crushed
- tsp dried oregano
- pinch ground turmeric

INSTRUCTIONS:

1. Heat oil in a large frying pan over high heat. Add mushroom . Cook, stirring, for 5 minutes or until golden and tender.
2. Add chilli , garlic , oregano and turmeric . Cook, stirring, for 1 minute or until fragrant. Season with salt and pepper. Serve.

LENTIL SOUP

INGREDIENTS:

- 2l vegetable or ham stock
- 150g red lentils
- 6 carrots, finely chopped
- 2 medium leeks, sliced (about 300g)
- small handful of chopped parsley, to serve

INSTRUCTIONS:

1. Heat the stock in a large pan and add the lentils. Bring to the boil and allow the lentils to soften for a few minutes.
2. Add the carrots and leeks, and season (don't add salt if you use ham stock as it will make it too salty). Bring to the boil, then

reduce the heat, cover and simmer for 45 mins-1 hr until the lentils have broken down. Scatter over the parsley and serve with buttered bread.

GARLIC AND THYME MUSHROOMS

INGREDIENTS:

- 400g button mushrooms
- 200g Swiss brown mushrooms, halved
- 2 garlic cloves, thinly sliced
- tbsp fresh thyme leaves
- tbsp olive oil
- 50g low-fat feta, crumbled

INSTRUCTIONS:

1. Preheat oven to 200°C/180°C fan-forced. Place mushroom, garlic, and thyme in a large baking dish. Drizzle with oil. Toss to combine.
2. Bake, stirring halfway through cooking, for 20 to 25 minutes or until mushrooms are tender and browned. Season with salt and pepper. Top with feta. Serve.

EGGPLANT, TOMATO AND PARSLEY SALAD WITH MINT YOGHURT DRESSING

INGREDIENTS:

- 2 eggplants, cut into 1cm-thick slices
- Olive oil spray
- 2 ripe tomatoes, finely chopped
- cup fresh continental parsley leaves

MINT YOGHURT DRESSING

- 70g (1/4 cup) skim milk natural yoghurt
- 2 tsp bought mint sauce
- tbsp chopped fresh mint
- tsp fresh lemon juice

INSTRUCTIONS:

1. To make dressing, combine the yoghurt, mint sauce, fresh mint and lemon juice in a jug. Season with salt and pepper.
2. Heat a barbecue grill on high. Lightly spray the eggplant with olive oil spray. Season with salt. Cook for 2 minutes each side or until brown and tender. Cut into 2cm strips.

3. Place the eggplant, tomato and parsley in a large bowl. Gently toss to combine.
4. Place the eggplant mixture on a serving plate and drizzle with the dressing. Serve.

VEGAN BANANA BREAD

INGREDIENTS:

- 3 large black bananas
- 75ml vegetable oil or sunflower oil, plus extra for the tin
- 100g brown sugar
- 225g plain flour (or use self-raising flour and reduce the baking powder to 2 heaped tsp)
- 3 heaped tsp baking powder
- 3 tsp cinnamon or mixed spice
- 50g dried fruit or nuts (optional)

INSTRUCTIONS:

1. Heat oven to 200C/180C fan/gas 6. Mash 3 large black peeled bananas with a fork, then mix well with 75g vegetable or sunflower oil and 100g brown sugar.

2. Add 225g plain flour, 3 heaped tsp baking powder and 3 tsp cinnamon or mixed spice, and combine well. Add 50g dried fruit or nuts, if using.
3. Bake in an oiled, lined 2lb loaf tin for 20 minutes. Check and cover with foil if the cake is browning.
4. Bake for another 20 minutes, or until a skewer comes out clean.
5. Allow to cool a little before slicing. It's delicious freshly baked, but develops a lovely gooey quality the day after.

LAMB AND ALMOND RICE PILAF

INGREDIENTS:

- 1/2 tbsp olive oil
- 1 brown onion, finely chopped
- garlic cloves, crushed
- 1 tbsp boiling water
- Pinch of saffron threads
- 625ml (2 1/2 cups) Massel salt reduced chicken style liquid stock
- 1 x 7cm cinnamon stick

- 300g (1 1/2 cups) Basmati rice
- 25g (1/4 cup) flaked almonds
- 200g cup mushrooms, thinly sliced
- 400g lamb eye of loin (backstrap)
- 1 bunch asparagus, woody ends trimmed, cut into 2cm pieces
- 150g (1 cup) frozen peas
- ripe tomatoes, coarsely chopped
- 1/4 cup chopped fresh continental parsley

INSTRUCTIONS:

1. Heat 1 tablespoon of oil in a large saucepan over medium heat. Add the onion and garlic and cook, stirring occasionally, for 4 minutes or until the onion softens.
2. Meanwhile, combine the water and saffron in a small bowl. Place the stock and cinnamon in a medium saucepan over medium heat. Bring to a simmer.
3. Add rice to the onion mixture. Cook, stirring, for 2 minutes. Add the saffron mixture and the stock mixture. Bring to a simmer. Reduce heat to low. Cover and cook, without stirring, for 12 minutes.

4. While the rice is cooking, place the almonds in a large frying pan over medium heat and cook, stirring, for 3 minutes or until toasted. Transfer to a large plate. Heat the remaining oil in the frying pan over medium-high heat. Add the mushroom and cook for 4 minutes or until tender. Transfer to the plate with the almonds. Add the lamb to the pan and cook for 3 minutes each side for medium or until cooked to your liking. Transfer to the plate.
5. Add asparagus , peas and tomato to the rice. Set aside, covered, for 5 minutes.
6. Thickly slice the lamb across the grain. Add the lamb, almonds, mushroom and parsley to the rice mixture and combine. Season with salt and pepper to serve.

SPRING FRUIT SALAD

INGREDIENTS:

- 5 large pink grapefruit
- cup white sugar
- 1 vanilla bean

- 1.3kg seedless watermelon
- Red Delicious apples
- 400g red grapes, removed from stalks
- x 250g punnets strawberries, sliced

INSTRUCTIONS:

1. Juice 1 grapefruit. Combine sugar and 1/2 cup grapefruit juice in a small saucepan. Cut vanilla bean through centre, leaving bean connected at base. Scrape soft black seeds out of centre. Add seeds and bean to sugar mixture. Stir over low heat for 5 minutes or until sugar has dissolved and syrup just comes to the boil. Reduce heat to low. Simmer, without stirring, for 5 minutes. Remove from heat. Allow to cool completely.
2. Using a knife, remove skin and pith from remaining 4 grapefruit. Cut into wedges. Remove skin from watermelon. Cut flesh into 2cm cubes. Cut apples into quarters. Remove cores and discard. Dice apple.

3. Arrange watermelon in a large serving bowl. Top with grapes, apples, grapefruit and strawberries. Drizzle with syrup. Serve.

BALSAMIC BEEF WITH GREEN BEANS AND MASH

INGREDIENTS;

- 1kg orange sweet potato (kumara), peeled, cut into 2cm pieces
- tsp olive oil
- 4 beef fillet steaks, excess fat trimmed
- 125ml (1/2 cup) balsamic vinegar
- 60ml (1/4 cup) Massel beef stock
- 60ml (1/4 cup) water
- 8 corn cobbettes
- 250g green beans, topped

INSTRUCTIONS:

1. Place the sweet potato in a large saucepan and cover with cold water. Bring to the boil over high heat and cook for 10 minutes or until tender. Drain and use a potato masher

or fork to mash until smooth. Season with pepper.

2. Meanwhile, heat the oil in a large non-stick frying pan over medium-high heat. Add the steaks and cook for 2-3 minutes each side for medium or until cooked to your liking. Transfer to a plate and cover loosely with foil. Set aside for 5 minutes to rest. Add the vinegar, stock and water to the pan. Bring to the boil over high heat. Boil, uncovered, for 6-7 minutes or until the mixture reduces and thickens slightly.
3. While the sauce is cooking, place the corn in a steamer basket over saucepan of simmering water. Steam, covered, for 5 minutes. Add the green beans to the basket with the corn and steam, covered, for a further 4 minutes or until the vegetables are just tender.
4. Divide the sweet potato mash among serving plates. Top with the steak and drizzle over the balsamic sauce. Serve with the steamed corn and green beans.

HONEY MUSTARD OCEAN TROUT WITH ROCKET AND ORANGE SALAD

INGREDIENTS:

- 4 (180g each) ocean trout fillets, skin removed
- 2 tbsp dijon mustard
- tbsp honey
- large oranges
- 1 tbsp apple cider vinegar
- tsp olive oil
- 80g rocket
- 1/2 cup pitted kalamata olives

INSTRUCTIONS:

1. Preheat grill on high heat. Line a baking tray with baking paper. Place fish on tray. Whisk mustard and honey together in a bowl. Reserve 1 tablespoon of mixture. Brush trout with remaining mustard mixture. Cook under grill for 5 to 7 minutes or until light golden and just cooked through. Remove to a plate. Cover with foil to keep warm.

2. Meanwhile, peel and segment oranges over a bowl, reserving 1 tablespoon of juice. Whisk reserved juice, vinegar, oil and reserved mustard mixture together in a bowl.
3. Combine rocket, olives, orange segments and dressing in a bowl. Serve fish with rocket and orange salad.

Printed in Great Britain
by Amazon

16992285R00071